Definitive Kettlebell Guide:

For The Versatility One

Richard Robertson

Introduction

Kettlebells are still relatively new to the fitness industry. Along with the barbell and dumbbell, they are amongst many machines designed to do one or two exercises. However, the kettlebell has been around for centuries with hidden benefits we have been tapping into for the past two decades. This guide is designed to give you all the information needed to understand its origins, versatility of use, and how to implement it for all goals desired. You will come to find that for being one simple object, there is a lot you can do with it.

Understanding the kettlebell is important. It is easy to use for someone just starting their fitness journey, yet is also quite useful for athletes and advanced lifters. Everyone would like to be healthy and fit, but it can be intimidating to have to commit to a gym and figure out how to use all of the different equipment. It is confusing and daunting to enter a gym and perform unfamiliar movements in front of strangers. Kettlebells help you understand your body and can easily be used anywhere with little space. Do you want to get stronger and lose fat? Improve your overall quality of life with minimal investment? Then this simple object was meant for your hands to grip and move.

Table of Contents

The History of the Kettlebell

"Never contest for space with a kettlebell." - Pavel Tsatsouline

Greek Halteres, Russian Girya, and now the kettlebell. All terms for a simple piece of equipment used to create strength champions from ancient Olympics to modern-day athletes. Credit goes mainly to Russia for the use of kettlebells as a body strengthening tool that led to competitive use as well. The culmination of centuries of existence led to its full-blown use for physical training in the early 21st century in the United States. Let us take a deeper look into the unique history of the kettlebell, and why it has become an established "new" type of equipment for the American population to use for strength and full-body training.

Although Russia holds the credit, the use of equipment similar to the kettlebell dates back to ancient Greek history, one of the first civilizations to incorporate resistance training for physical development and sport training. The well-known concept of progressive overload dates back to ancient Greece, which gives you an understanding of how useful this equipment has been to make it through to our modern-day society. The Scotland Highland Games have weighted objects with a handle that can be swung, which demonstrates the use of a kettlebell-like object that has changed overtime. Just like a car, equipment for lifting updates over time to be more efficient and effective.

Germany should also be given credit for the use of kettlebells as part of a strength training program. Many diaries, journals, and other historical documents discuss the use of kettlebells for strength performance. Strongman competitions were quite popular and date back to the 18th and 19th centuries, before the use of the kettlebell as an accepted exercise in Russia. Instead, the earliest documents in Russian history discussing the kettlebell only indicate its use by farmers as a counterweight for grains. Eventually, farmers began to use it to pass time and demonstrate strength. As international travel became popular, the well-known doctor Vladislav Krayevsky attended a German strongman competition that used this object for sporting events and training.

Two years later he wrote about how the kettlebell is important for sports medicine and informed the Russian Czar of his findings. Later this would be a required training protocol for the Russian army, recommended for citizens to use to reduce health costs, and eventually turned into a popular sport. This is one reason Russian weightlifters dominated their sport since they had already popularized kettlebell use prior to, which encouraged the use of full-body resistance training to encourage both strength and power.

Pavel Tsatsouline, Soviet Union special forces instructor, later migrated to the United States in the '90s. He is accredited with the introduction of the kettlebell for physical conditioning in America. He later developed a kettlebell workout program to help Americans understand how to use the equipment and put together a training program. However, even though Pavel gets the credit, the use of the kettlebell for athletic conditioning was actually seen in America during the early 1900s.

Kettlebell and strongman athletes that migrated from Russia and Germany brought their knowledge with them and started showing men in the gym what they had learned. Many coaches and gym owners were immigrants from these areas known to use the kettlebell. Somewhere in the mid-1900s, use of the kettlebell declined, most likely due to World War Two taking place and the focus on physical fitness taking a backseat to other concerns.

Modern-day society now fully embraces that kettlebells have a lot to offer in terms of conditioning, versatility, and overall health benefits. However, too many fear it as an advanced piece of equipment that is difficult to use, or they simply have trained for so long without it they do not really know what exactly to do with this odd-shaped object. The main reason people do not allow something new into their lives is because it is unfamiliar and they fear looking awkward and not knowing how to use it correctly. The purpose of this guide is to first educate you on the use of the kettlebell, as knowledge is power, and then teach you how to apply the use of this equipment effectively to any workout program to achieve any goal.

Benefits of Kettlebell Training

What a disgrace it is for a man to grow old without ever seeing the beauty and strength of which his body is capable." - Socrates

There are many benefits to be derived from using the kettlebell as a training tool. Athletes from ancient to modern day would not be where they were without this type of equipment being incorporated into their training programs. The key points that differentiate kettlebell training from dumbbell and barbell training are:

- Full Body Conditioning Tool
- Enhances Body Awareness and Coordination
- Mixture of Strength, Power, and Cardio
- Improves Posture, Imbalances, and Muscle Weaknesses
- Easy to Train Anywhere and Ease of Storage

The dumbbell is the only free-weight piece of equipment that resembles the kettlebell, but the design differences are what separate them from each other. The dumbbell is very one-sided in terms of design: a simple straight line with equal weight at the ends. Basically, the dumbbell has already balanced the resistance out for you to easily operate. Physical conditioning was not meant to be easy, and the difficulty of movement is what uses more muscle groups and strength to overcome the imbalance the kettlebell provides.

Simply put, the kettlebell is a solid ball with a handle attached on top. Almost all the resistance is within the ball, which distributes the weight on this center of focus, allowing gravity to naturally make the kettlebell highly effective.

The basics are what truly still work. There are too many unnecessary isolation movements being created with resistance pulley cables, but not many frequent gym enthusiasts are incorporating the kettlebell into their workout. The equipment is readily there as coaches and gym owners know they are important to have, but many walk by the kettlebell with only side glances, scared to try something new.

Isolation seems to be what many consider the correct way to perform a workout, but in reality, you want to accomplish more from your training program within a specified time frame. Your body can only handle so much stress before fatigue sets in and muscle waste occurs. Targeting multiple muscle groups is the key to seeing results in both strength and muscle development.

Full Body Conditioning Tool

The kettlebell targets the body as a whole during training. You can use the equipment for isolation like a dumbbell, but this would defeat the purpose of such a unique tool for conditioning. The reason your body is used as a whole is that both larger muscle groups and stabilizer muscles need to be activated to execute a movement. The kettlebell swing is a great example and a fundamental exercise to utilize.

When executing the movement, your body goes into a hinged position, which activates your posterior chain and tightens your core to swing the kettlebell forward. While your core remains tight, your upper body muscles continue the swing to stabilize at the point of completion. All this takes place from one single movement! Since you are using your body as a whole, your blood must pump oxygen to your muscles faster, thus encouraging a heightened heart rate, leading to cardio as well. More will be covered about specific exercises later in your reading, but the point is that a single exercise can condition your body fully. Consider what multiple exercises would do for your training program.

Enhances Body Awareness and Coordination

Proprioception: Awareness of the position and movement of the body. This is basically your ability to be coordinated in how you move and balance yourself to prevent falling over. The concept "mind to muscle connection" also ties into body awareness since you need to understand how your muscles move dynamically i.e. constant changes from one area to another. During kettlebell training, you swing toward your sides, up over your head, down between your legs, and even go from the floor to the standing position for a few exercises.

The need to be completely focused is imperative to execute the exercises safely and effectively. Will you have full understanding the first time you use a kettlebell? Probably not. Kettlebells require hands-on training just like anything else to improve your movement and understand how your body reacts to the dynamic changes of the resistance in different directions. This makes it impossible to jump straight into a heavy kettlebell workout. Muscle and strength need to develop progressively, and over time you will have to modify your resistance accordingly to ensure the body can change with your goals.

Mixture of Strength, Cardio, and Power

The kettlebell is a superior training tool because it mixes all planes of training into your exercises: strength and muscle, cardio, and power. Strength training is moving your body against resistance to make it stronger. Your body cannot move without the use of your muscles, thus the reason "muscle building" doesn't need to be its own separate category. Strength development will allow muscles to grow and increase in muscular endurance.

Strength does not just pertain to how your muscles grow, or how much weight you can swing around. This type of training is also imperative for you to be healthy and for joints to function properly. Even those in their senior years are required to perform some type of strength training for 120 minutes per week for a better quality of life. Why? Because bones become stronger when you train against resistance. The human body is very adaptable to its environment, and if your bones are placed under controlled pressure, the cells will signal increased development. Not everyone is the same, but studies prove that bones will get stronger than they previously were.

Cardiovascular training is performing exercises that activate the aerobic pathway, which is when your body requires oxygen to produce energy referred to as ATP. While your blood pumps the oxygen into your body for energy, your heart rate increases, requiring you to control your breathing and encouraging your heart to grow stronger. After the glucose (sugar) in your muscle stores have been used up, your body will do a metabolic switch to burn fat as fuel instead. Those not used to this will experience lightheadedness due to the lack of glucose and increased oxygen flow. Cardio-based strength training is progressive with intensity just like increasing the resistance. Ease into the intensity and allow your body to adapt instead of being in complete shock.

Power increases as a result of kettlebell training as well. Strength and power are often thought to be the same, but this is not true since they both have their own specific way of utilizing force. Power is the ability to apply the speed of maximal force against a load, while strength is the maximal force you can place on the load. Speed through power is what encourages further full body use to create the momentum that moves the kettlebell against heavier loads.

Improves Posture, Imbalances, and Muscle Weaknesses

Full body movements with the kettlebell can even improve factors such as balance and your posture. Through the use of your core and stabilizer muscles, you are able to strengthen muscles that normally are not activated through other types of resistance training. Since several movements require your body to be hinged at the hips, the posterior chain is strengthened and will develop muscles that improve your posture. However, they will not completely fix issues such as kyphosis, which is the rounding of your upper back (aka hunchback). The kettlebell corrects many issues and provides numerous benefits, but it's not a magical device.

A weak core is one of the main reasons why you would feel imbalanced and hard to get your center of gravity. Your core is not just your abdominal muscles; it is a group of muscles that work together to protect your spine and provide balance. Essentially, it is the muscles that attach to your spinal column or pelvis.

Muscles included are:

- Rectus and Transversus Abdominis
- Internal and External Obliques
- Spinal Erectors and Multidus
- Latissimus Dorsi and Trapezius
- Adductors and Glutes
- Diaphragm

You can see your core is much more than just your abs and lower back. Many of the muscle groups apply to your posterior chain, which is why having a strong back and legs is what keeps your body healthy even into your senior years. Olympic weightlifters and those that perform CrossFit execute training programs that teach the use of their core and develop it fully. Kettlebells are one of the dynamic tools that make this possible.

Many fitness enthusiasts have a weak core and no understanding of how to activate these muscles to brace for a movement. The appearance of abdominal muscles does not mean a person has a strong core either. A great example would be those that compete in the strongman competition. They usually do not have a flat stomach with "shredded abs," but rather a solid, round stomach. There would be no way for them to move the loads they do without a strong core.

Pure strength truly only takes you so far until injury occurs. Stereotypes that focus on appearance over health plague the fitness industry. The reality is that if you focus on getting stronger and encouraging a better lifestyle change, then your body will appear aesthetically better as well. The lean muscle appearance has a lot to do with your diet over exercise.

Kettlebells are Convenient

One of the best features of the kettlebell is that it is convenient. Convenient for storage, training space, and even time as well. A full kettlebell workout can be completed in only 20-30 minutes depending on the intensity yet will give you more benefits than a 60-90 minute workout using machines. The ability to conserve the amount of time needed for a workout gives you little reason to not train, and no travel would even be needed if you prefer home training.

You do not need an entire rack of dumbbells taking up space. Usually 2-3 kettlebells of varying resistances are all that are needed.

Less equipment means less storage space, as they can easily be placed into the corner of a room or the garage.

Who Can Use Kettlebells?

This type of equipment is nearly universal in use. Studies show that with supervision and proper training, even children as young as six can benefit from Olympic weightlifting. The point is not to lift heavy loads, but rather to develop a habit of being active and strengthening the body as it grows. Learning proper coordination and use of their body carries over significantly as they get older. The same even applies to those in their senior years. An overhead squat is an amazing exercise for functional training. Again, this does not require a heavy weight. The movements with kettlebells are similar in using the entire body to move the weight, thus improving the joints and their ability to functionally move.

The answer to who can use kettlebells is essentially everyone medically cleared to perform physical activities. Strength training is not something to skip out on, and most doctors these days recommend it, as opposed to only cardio or walking on a treadmill. Some may have restrictions on the amount of weight that can be used or have a specific heart rate they need to stay within. A qualified personal trainer or strength coach should be consulted to execute the workout and ensure safety if this applies to you, a family member, or friend.

Many who participate in kettlebell training started off with bad joint mobility such as in the hips and shoulders. Slight pain may be experienced at first, which is normal in the case of a previous injury with scar tissue surrounding the joint. However, through functional training with the kettlebell, joint mobility has the possibility of improving drastically. Those barely capable of lifting their arms parallel to the floor can now do so naturally without pain, and others have improved their shoulder mobility to reach overhead as well. You can utilize kettlebell training routinely for your health and physical changes no matter your age or gender.

Different Training Variations

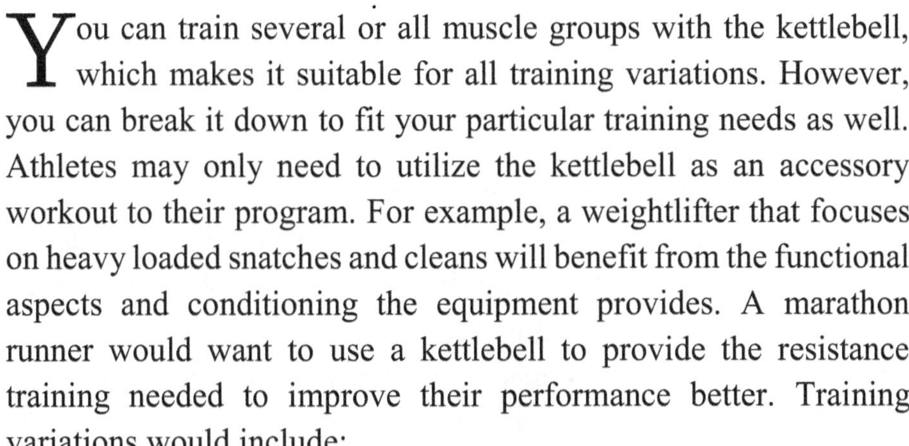

You can train several or all muscle groups with the kettlebell, which makes it suitable for all training variations. However, you can break it down to fit your particular training needs as well. Athletes may only need to utilize the kettlebell as an accessory workout to their program. For example, a weightlifter that focuses on heavy loaded snatches and cleans will benefit from the functional aspects and conditioning the equipment provides. A marathon runner would want to use a kettlebell to provide the resistance training needed to improve their performance better. Training variations would include:

- Cross Training
- Functional Training
- Speed and Endurance
- Strength Training

These primary focuses work best for kettlebell use under specific circumstances. Isolation is not necessary when utilizing a strength training program. Muscles will develop from the exercises and allow growth throughout the body with proper programming. The only time it is necessary to do specific muscle isolation is for improper growth or weaker muscles. For example, one leg that is growing more than the other may require more single leg movements to offset the load to each leg.

Cross Training

Cross training applies to a wider variety of training methods, but the overall goal is improving on your current weaknesses. Essentially, you are trying to break a routine to bypass doing the same exercises every week. The ones who benefit from this specific type of training are athletes, or if you have intermediate to advanced experience in physical training. Constant training toward your specific competitive goals is still needed for powerlifting and weightlifting, but after a certain time frame you may start to just maintain your progress.

This is called a plateau. You essentially see little to no changes in your body and performance. Change in your routine is needed to overcome the habit your muscles have developed. The human body will adapt to a constant routine for survival, and if you do the same lifts and workouts every week, eventually you will not get any further results. Plus, boredom with the routine can cause people to become lazy. Some may even want to give up or switch sports since they see no further progress. However, cross training can easily be the solution for this common issue.

Exercises for cross training will vary for your individual goals. For example, powerlifters execute heavy loaded movements with simple yet powerful exercises such as squats, bench, and deadlifts. The old method for training was just pure raw strength. Mass moves mass. Previous strength athletes were very stiff and lacked mobility in the powerlifting world. Now, we see men and women with amazing physiques capable of lifting much more, especially those in their younger years.

Why? The focus on mobility, flexibility, and accessory exercises for weaknesses have been incorporated. Proper use of cross training can alleviate injuries, especially in the hips and shoulders. The big three lifts are still an area of focus, but the additional movements for cross training can enhance performance and progress.

Functional Training

Functional training is the execution of movements that strengthen your body to carry over to everyday life. The ability to sit and stand from a chair or toilet. Having the strength to get yourself off the floor without injury, or simply being able to reach for an item on the top shelf. These are all movements that are essential for day-to-day life. Many suffer from ailments that prevent them from doing even the most basic of movements due to age, prior injury, and the most common reason: lack of physical activities.

Functional movements can be those that mimic daily life such as squats and deadlifts, or simply exercises that strengthen your body for these movements. The whole point for exercising at the end of the day is to prepare your body for activities beyond the workout.

It's no coincidence that kettlebell training carries over to everyday life with the use of compound movements. Compound movements use multiple muscle groups to accomplish an exercise, and these are the primary uses for functional training. Extra exercises performed are lunges, kettlebell swings, and the clean and press. This is not to take away from physical activities such as cable pull downs and the dumbbell press. Being physically active is always important and holds benefits. However, the kettlebell simply does more for your body within a shorter time frame.

Speed and Endurance

Several kettlebell exercises help improve your speed and endurance. The ballistic nature of the kettlebell helps produce explosive power throughout the body. This quick explosiveness increases your speed and ability to react quicker with better control. Speed training with kettlebells can be exercises such as the snatch, cleans, kettlebell swings, and jerk variations. The ability to execute an exercise with explosiveness is a primary necessity for kettlebell use. Cardio training derives from this as well due to the intensity needed as the repetitions start taking place.

Usually people expect cardio to come from high rep counts and/or supersets. However, just one speed-based movement performed for 12 repetitions can increase cardio after 3-4 sets with minimal rest times between. Your muscles develop endurance this way through the constant need to stabilize your body, produce power, and control the resistance. Having endurance assists with many situations such as athletes needing to perform for long durations, or simply walking from your car to the grocery store. Either situation requires using your muscles to get around, regardless of intensity.

Strength Training

Strength training doesn't mean you need a ridiculously large kettlebell where you only perform a few repetitions with it. Instead, you can use the same kettlebell weight for many exercises with controlled repetitions. Yes, this does mean the kettlebell will be slightly lighter than the one you throw over your head, but the purpose is to have just a few options. Why lighter instead of heavier resistance? Ballistic movements like swings use explosive technique instead of controlled. Exercises that are not ballistic are classified as "grinds," which are slower in execution and more focused.

Essentially there is no momentum during strength training. There really is no need to have numerous kettlebells, though. Just 2-3 different resistances should be more than enough. The purpose of a strength training program is to help perform movements that target muscle regions and control the exercises to activate more muscles.

Strength is going to come from any type of these training variations. However, being able to control the resistance effectively assists with producing better strength potential. Even resistance bands can be utilized for these moderately intense exercises. For example, the goblet squat focuses on your lower body, hips, and core muscles. A resistance band can be attached to the handle with the kettlebell being held upside down. This will help force more stabilizer muscles to become activated while overcoming the resistance from the pull of the band.

Exercises that are based on strength rather than cardio or speed are single leg deadlifts, floor presses, and alternating shoulder presses. You can see these movements lack the intensity and momentum and can be performed with slightly lighter resistance. This is the training style most beginners and seniors would want to focus on for their starting kettlebell program. The main reason is for getting used to the movement and control of your body with a kettlebell prior to ballistic movements, aside from swings. Developing grip strength helps reduce the possibility of injuring your wrists during exercises like the snatch or clean.

Choosing the Right Kettlebell

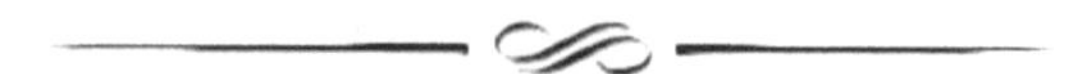

The only time anything really applies to opposite genders is the amount of resistance chosen for the kettlebell. Testosterone is the dominant male hormone that allows men to have stronger bones and develop strength faster. Does this mean women can't be strong? Absolutely not. This just means that a male who is inactive or a beginner will naturally be able to use a higher resistance level than a female starting out. When couples start training together, the amount of resistance is relatively the same. After a few months of equal work, the male will generally surpass the female's resistance level.

However, the downfall of this inequality is two-sided. Men will aim for a heavier resistance, especially if they are already used to strength training. The bad part of this is that the body will not be used for controlled movements that require balance and control. Overstraining the stabilizer muscles that have never really been used can cause injury. Similarly, some women starting out will pick up a kettlebell and automatically state it is too heavy. Accommodating the needs to your kettlebell choosing needs to be with an open mindset to prevent wasting money.

This is good to keep in mind if you plan to be a strength training coach. Resistance (weight) to choose for your kettlebell depends on a few factors:

- Resistance Training Level and Experience
- Age, Weight, Gender
- Ballistic or Grind

Taking these factors into account, the following resistances are the most common for their specified categories with beginners:

Male Beginner

Ballistic Exercises – 14kg(30lbs) – 20kg(44lbs)

Grind Exercises – 8kg(18lbs) – 12kg(26lbs)

Female Beginner

Ballistic Exercises – 8kg(18lbs) – 12kg(26lbs)

Grind Exercises – 4kg(9lbs) – 8kg(18lbs)

The first kettlebell resistance is recommended for those beginners with little to no experience doing physical activities. The higher end of the resistance levels is for those new to kettlebells with some experience doing resistance training. However, if you are athletic and new to kettlebells, you may need to be hands on with your choosing and try the heaviest resistance for beginners first. After a couple of sets, it may be necessary to go the next size up. Those very weak or in their senior years may want the next kettlebell size down from the first resistance shown.

Kettlebell training is not based on progressive overload on a weekly or bi-weekly basis. The point of a kettlebell and the specific exercises utilized for training limits the need to progressively increase your resistance. Kettlebells vary in size and shape as well. Some brands will have thin handles and a not very round-shaped bell, while others have thicker handles and not much room to fit both hands for two-handed swings.

The easiest solution is purchasing competition-based kettlebells to ensure good size, handle width, and proper design. This will enable a smoother flow to your movements. If you are only able to find a smaller kettlebell, you can still make use of it, although some exercises may not be able to be performed until a kettlebell with a wider grip becomes available.

Fundamental Kettlebell Exercises

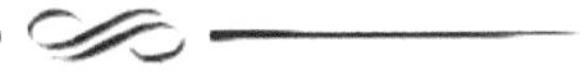

Now it's time to actually learn the basic fundamentals for kettlebell exercises. There are many different exercises to choose from when it comes to training, but the ones presented here are kettlebell specific and not really ones you would execute with a dumbbell and most certainly not a barbell. You will be given a step-by-step guide on how to safely and successfully execute each exercise.

Most specific movements to cover are ballistic based. Several exercises are similar to what you would execute with a dumbbell as well, but good to know for a training program. Plus, using a kettlebell makes the exercises slightly more difficult with the weight not evenly distributed. The intent is to learn how to utilize your body as a whole to stabilize, balance, and create ballistic explosions when needed. Proper technique and form are as must!

Unilateral Training

Unilateral training is one method of training that you have to understand before learning about kettlebell exercises. This type of training is when you use weight on only one side of your body. This is one of the main reasons why kettlebell training is so beneficial for your body to develop and get stronger. The best way to get your core muscles activated is by forcing them to counter the weight pulling your body to one side.

When the load pulls in one direction, your stabilizer muscles and core react to keep you from falling over. This method helps a lot when it comes to balance work and you are also getting strength and muscle development as well. Balance-based exercises don't normally do this and require a balance pad to be utilized. Extra equipment like that really is not needed when you simply perform many of the different kettlebell exercises with one hand.

Double and Single Hand Swings

Type: Ballistic

Primary Focus: Shoulders, Back, Core, Hips, Quads, Hamstrings

Execution (Two Hand):

1. Place the kettlebell arm's length in front of you on the floor, standing with feet shoulder width apart.

2. Bend at the hips and grasp the kettlebell with both hands on the handle, palms down and arms fully extended.

3. When ready, pull the kettlebell, keeping a hinge in your hips and a straight lower back to swing the kettlebell back between your legs.

4. Keeping your arms extended the entire execution, push your hips forward as you swing the kettlebell forward until body is standing tall, and the kettlebell is parallel with the floor.

5. Bend at your hips as gravity takes the kettlebell back down to repeat the movement.

The one-handed swing is executed the same way but holding the handle with one hand, allowing your trunk to slightly twist inward naturally to allow swing range of motion.

Advanced Method: Swings can be made slightly more difficult as well. You can alternate hands each time you swing the kettlebell up to standing position. Also, gripping tightly and maintaining arms fully extended, you can take the swing range of motion fully overhead for better shoulder rotation and core activation. Again, these are advanced movements and should not be executed until regular swings have been learned properly.

Clean

Cleans are the second most needed exercise to master and get used to. Many exercises are based on cleaning into the racked position before even executing the movement. The "racked" position is a basic fundamental for kettlebell exercises. This is when you hold the kettlebell aligned with your shoulder(s) with your hand in front and close to the chest. The kettlebell will rest across the forearm within the pocket(s) your elbow and upper arm form.

Type: Ballistic

Primary Focus: Shoulders, Back, Core, Quads, Hamstrings

Execution:

- **NOTE: From this point on, if an exercise starts with the instructions to clean the kettlebell up into the racked position, you will execute the entire exercise pattern steps 1-3.**

1. Place the kettlebell between your feet on the floor, standing with feet shoulder width apart.

2. Partially hinge over the kettlebell, keeping your chest up, and grasp the kettlebell palm down and arm fully extended.

3. Explode pushing your feet into the ground, driving your hips forward, and flicking your wrist to rotate the kettlebell into the racked position.

4. Allow gravity to rotate the kettlebell back into the previous position, simultaneously controlling the resistance down to extend your arm and swing between your legs.

5. Repeat by using the momentum coming forward from the swing to pull back up into the racked position.

An alternative method is after cleaning the kettlebell into the racked position, you can allow the weight to swing down and control back to the floor. Either method is fine and mainly depends on the intensity you desire and the resistance chosen.

Double and Single Racked Squats

Type: Grind

Primary Focus: Quads, Hamstrings, Hips, Core

Execution (One Handed):

1. Grasp the kettlebell and clean into the racked position standing with your body fully upright and feet shoulder width apart.

2. Extend the non-loaded arm out from the body to create balance.

3. Tighten your core by bracing from taking a breath into your diaphragm.

4. Simultaneously bend at your hips and knees, dropping into the squat position.

5. Try to not lean for countering the offset loading, dropping minimum depth of hips parallel with the floor.

6. Drive your feet down, pushing your body back up into the starting position.

Two-handed racked squats are executed the same way, but instead you are now holding a kettlebell in each hand. Core is still strengthened this way, but not as much emphasis as with a single kettlebell. Plus, it is cost efficient to not buy two kettlebells the same weight. However, the choice is yours depending on your budget and preference.

Clean & Jerk

Type: Ballistic

Primary Focus: Shoulders, Back, Core, Quads, Hamstrings

Execution:

1. Grasp the kettlebell and clean into the racked position, standing with your body fully upright and feet shoulder width apart.

2. From the racked position, partially bend at your knees and explode, allowing feet to slightly rise from the floor and go out to form a stable base.

3. Simultaneously while your lower body is exploding, your palm is being driven up to fully extend your arm overhead using the leg drive to complete as fast as possible.

4. Lower the kettlebell back into the racked position. From this point, go back into the clean starting position and repeat the steps to jerk again.

An alternative to this exercise is performing a split jerk. This is when you throw the opposite leg out in front of you during the explosion, which is exactly what Olympic weightlifters do. However, the difference is if using one hand, you will want to throw out the leg that is opposite the load bearing side. For example, if the kettlebell is in your right hand, you will throw your left foot forward.

Push Press

The push press strongly resembles the normal jerk, but instead of exploding, you are simply bending at your knees to use leg drive for the press. This allows you to take strain off the shoulder to perform higher resistance or more repetitions.

Type: Ballistic

Primary Focus: Shoulders, Upper Back, Core

Execution:

1. Grasp the kettlebell and clean into the racked position, standing with your body fully upright and feet shoulder width apart.

2. Slightly bend at your knees as if performing a partial squat.

3. Drive your feet down and extend your legs fully.

4. Simultaneously, your palm is driving up with the leg drive until the arm is fully extended.

5. Return back to the racked position while partially squatting to take the impact of the resistance coming down, and then repeat to execute more repetitions.

Snatch

This is a more advanced exercise. Ensure that you learn how to properly clean prior to performing a snatch. Cleans help develop your wrist and forearm strength and get you familiar with the feeling of the kettlebell rotating into your lower arm.

Type: Ballistic

Primary Focus: Shoulders, Back, Core, Hips, Quads, Hamstrings

Execution:

1. Place the kettlebell arm's length in front of you on the floor, standing with feet shoulder width apart.

2. Bend at the hips and grasp the kettlebell with both hands on the handle, palms down and arms fully extended.

3. When ready, pull the kettlebell, keeping a hinge in your hips and a straight lower back to swing the kettlebell back between your legs.

4. As the swing comes forward, you will trace your body into an upright row.

5. Simultaneously, while rowing the kettlebell up, you begin to rotate your lower arm to allow the kettlebell to swing to the front of your forearm as you extend your arm fully overhead.

6. Lock your shoulder and elbow to fully complete the exercise.

7. Control back down into the swinging position between your legs and repeat.

Windmill

Type: Grind

Primary Focus: Shoulders, Core, Hips, Hamstrings

Execution:

1. Go into the racked position and push the kettlebell overhead. Maintain this position with your arm fully extended overhead for the movement.

2. Keeping your eyes locked onto the kettlebell, begin lowering

your body, reaching for the floor with your opposite hand.

3. Opposite hand will trace your leg down, hips will push to the weight-bearing side, the opposite leg will slightly bend more than the loaded side.

4. Continue until you reach the lowest point, or until the tips of your fingers can touch the floor.

5. Reverse the process back up into starting position.

Remember, your arm is going to stay fully extended the entire time. Keeping your eyes locked onto the kettlebell allows your core to remain tight and your shoulder to move naturally as the torso lowers down. Not keeping your eyes on the kettlebell will cause your shoulder to not rotate properly.

Slingshot

This is a great warm-up exercise, perfect for getting used to kettlebell movements. This teaches your body to adapt to the balance and core work required, while also learning the grip of the kettlebell and how to maneuver it.

Type: Ballistic

Primary Focus: Shoulders, Core

Execution:

1. Grasp the kettlebell with both hands palms down and arms extended fully down.

2. Stand with feet shoulder width apart to create a good foundation for balance.

3. Keeping your body upright throughout the exercise, swing to one side of your body, releasing with the opposite hand.

4. Allow the kettlebell to fully rotate around your waist and grab behind the back with the opposite hand.

5. Continue this for the set repetitions, then switch to the opposite direction, or switch each full rotation around the body.

Halo

Lighter resistance makes this a great warm-up for your shoulders. Heavier resistance activates the muscles surrounding your shoulders for strength and muscle development.

Type: Grind

Primary Focus: Shoulders, Upper Back, Core

Execution:

1. Grasp the kettlebell by the outside of the handles with the ball portion up.

2. Keep the kettlebell held this way close to your body and your hands in front of your chest.

3. Rotate the kettlebell to the left or right of your head, grasping with both hands throughout.

4. Allow the kettlebell to circle around your back into the starting position.

5. You can stay on one side first for a set, or alternate direction after each repetition for better coordination.

Turkish Get-Up

Type: Grind

Primary Focus: Shoulders, Core, Quads, Hamstrings

Execution:

1. Lie on the floor, grasping the kettlebell in one hand.

2. Extend the load-bearing arm out, keeping your eyes on the kettlebell. Don't push your shoulder forward! Naturally press out and keep your shoulder in socket.

3. Bring your foot in from the same side as the load-bearing arm and plant firmly onto the floor close to your glute. Opposite leg stays extended out.

4. Take your non-loaded hand and place toward the outside of your body while simultaneously pushing your torso up. Hips stay on the floor.

5. After sitting up, you rotate the non-loaded leg to foot down on the floor as you extend your hips up into a bridge.

6. Rotate your hips to allow the non-loaded leg to swing below. You will be in a kneeling position with both legs by this point.

7. Remove your palm from the floor and stand until the body is fully erect.

8. Reverse the process to get back into the starting position.

Single Arm Deadlift

Type: Grind

Primary Focus: Back, Core, Hips, Quads, Hamstring

Execution:

1. Grasp the kettlebell in one hand, holding down the center of your body and with feet shoulder width apart.

2. Keeping your arm extended fully and back straight, hinge at your hips and slightly bend at your knees.

3. Keep pushing your hips back and lowering your torso until you feel tightness in the hamstrings.

4. Drive your hips forward and stand back into the starting position.

You can perform this movement with two hands as well, but a heavier kettlebell may be needed to get better muscle activation.

Single Leg Deadlift

Type: Grind

Primary Focus: Core, Hips, Quads, Hamstrings

Execution:

1. Grasp the kettlebell with your arm extended at your side.

2. Stand on the same leg as the load-bearing side and take your opposite foot off the floor as if balancing with one leg.

3. Keeping your back straight, slightly bend at your knee and push your hips back.

4. Continue this bend, allowing the kettlebell to naturally make its way forward, keeping your arm extended throughout.

5. Once you feel tightness on the hamstring, push your hips forward and stand back tall.

If the balance remains difficult even with proper bracing, you can use your opposite toes to tap the floor when your balance begins to sway. You can also make this exercise more difficult for your core by holding the kettlebell in the opposite hand of the leg used.

Goblet Squat

Similar to racked squats, but the resistance is held by both hands, keeping it directly at the center of your body. Improves squat patterns and good for beginners learning balance and core bracing.

Type: Grind

Primary Focus: Core, Hips, Quads, Hamstrings

Execution:

1. Grasp the kettlebell by the outside of the handles with the ball portion up.

2. Keep the kettlebell close to your body and hold this position for the entire movement.

3. Simultaneously bend at your hips and knees to drop into the squat position.

4. Strive to at least squat to where your hips are parallel with the floor.

5. Drive your feet down and bring your hips forward to complete the squat.

If gripping the kettlebell by the handles is straining at first, you can hold by the bottom of the circle in your palms until grip and wrist strength improve.

Good Mornings

Type: Grind

Primary Focus: Core, Hips, Hamstrings

Execution:

1. Grasp the kettlebell with two hands and rotate behind the

middle of your upper back. Palms should face down for better grip and elbows should be forward.

2. Allow the kettlebell to rest on your upper back the entire movement. Feet should be shoulder width apart.

3. Keeping your back straight, begin by bending at your knees slightly and pushing your hips back into a hinged position.

4. Lower further into the hinge until you feel the tightness in your hamstrings.

5. Push your hips forward and back into the starting position.

Alternative method is standing with a wider foot stance. This will allow you to target your hamstrings and glutes with some more emphasis.

Racked Double Lunges

Double lunge means you perform a forward lunge first, and then come out and swing your foot back to execute a reverse lunge. That is one complete repetition opposed to separating the two variations on their own.

Type: Grind

Primary Focus: Core, Hips, Quads, Hamstrings

Execution:

1. Start off in the racked position with feet hip width apart.

2. Keeping your body upright, initiate by taking an exaggerated step forward with the leg the load is being held on.

3. Come out of the lunge and continuously bring that foot back into a reverse lunge.

4. Come back to the starting position to repeat the exercise.

You can improve grip strength by holding a kettlebell in each hand throughout the repetitions for both legs. The difficulty can be increased by using the opposite leg the load is being held on.

Bent Rows

Type: Grind

Primary Focus: Shoulders, Back, Core

Execution:

1. Grasp the kettlebell with one hand and leave the kettlebell extended down your side.

2. Hinge at your hips to create a 45 degree angle or more with your body and arm extended down.

3. Begin pulling the kettlebell in toward your body, keeping your wrist straight and elbow close to your body.

4. Try not to rotate your torso to assist with the pull.

5. Continue the row until your elbow is close to going behind the back.

6. Control the resistance fully down and repeat.

You can perform this exercise with two kettlebells if you have the same resistance available.

Floor Press

Type: Grind

Primary Focus: Chest, Shoulders, Core

Execution:

1. Lie down on your back with legs fully extended on the floor.

2. Grasp the kettlebell in one hand and extend your arm out from your body.

3. The opposite hand should be palms down on the floor to stabilize your body. Teach your mind to not rotate your torso to twist for assistance.

4. Lower the kettlebell down, bending at the elbow and opening your chest up.

5. Once your upper arm rests against the floor, allow one second to pass and press the kettlebell back up.

Keeping your legs fully extended forces you to activate your core and place better emphasis on your chest. If this is difficult, you can bring your knees up and place your feet on the floor.

Sit and Press

Type: Grind

Primary Focus: Shoulders, Core

Execution:

1. Lie on your back with legs fully extended on the floor.

2. Grasp the kettlebell in your hands at the base and rest it in front of your chest.

3. Ensuring that your grip is tight, activate your core to sit up while simultaneously pressing the kettlebell up.

4. End point will be sitting up with the kettlebell pressed fully overhead. Legs stay extended the entire movement.

Straight Arm Sit-Up

Type: Grind

Primary Focus: Shoulders, Core

Execution:

1. Lie on your back with legs fully extended on the floor.

2. Grasp the kettlebell in one hand and extend your arm fully out.

3. Holding this position, tighten your core and sit up fully.

4. Your legs will stay extended on the floor the entire time.

5. Ending point will be when you sit fully up and your arm is extended overhead.

Farmers Carry

Type: Grind

Primary Focus: Shoulders, Back, Core

Execution:

1. Stand with the kettlebell held down at your side.

2. Initiate the exercise by simply walking the desired distance chosen.

3. Arm must remain extended down your side. Prevent your body from leaning to hold the resistance.

4. Switch sides and walk the same distance.

Kettlebell Workout Program: Full Body Strength Training

This kettlebell workout is focused primarily on grind-based exercises to help improve strength. Also, this would be a better starter workout for those learning how to utilize a kettlebell for training. Each exercise that's not ballistic-based should be performed with controlled motions. Doing so will help prevent injuries and allow better muscle activation. Grip strength will improve drastically for beginners with little impact to the wrists.

Program Key: 4x10-12 = 4 sets with 10 or 12 repetitions per set. 30-60 seconds max rest between each set.

Warm Up (Light Resistance):

A1 Slingshots – 2x8 (per side)

B1 Halos – 2x8 (per side)

C1 Windmill – 2x8 (per side)

Workout:

Each exercise is performed with given rest time between sets. Complete all sets before advancing to the next exercise. If a resistance feels slightly light, you can change the repetition range to 12-15 instead.

A1 Cleans – 3x10-12 (per side)

B1 Push Press - 3x10-12 (per side)

C1 Goblet Squats - 4x10-12

D1 Single Arm Deadlift - 3x10-12 (per side)

E1 Two-Handed Swings - 5x10-12

Kettlebell Workout Program: Full Body Conditioning

Conditioning is activating your muscles to build up endurance and prepare your body to train harder for more intense workouts. This program will be a mixture of single exercises and supersets as well. A superset is when you perform an exercise and then immediately perform the next exercise that uses opposing primary muscle groups. Although all exercises use similar muscles, the main focus isn't always the same. A superset will be noted with a letter followed by the number 2. For example, A1 then A2 means they will be grouped together with the same letter.

Program Key: 4x10-12 = 4 sets with 10 or 12 repetitions per set. 30-60 seconds max rest between each set. Supersets should only be a max rest of 15 seconds before executing the next exercise to complete the full set.

Warm Up (Light Resistance):

A1 Slingshots – 2x8 (per side)

B1 Halos – 2x8 (per side)

C1 Windmill – 2x8 (per side)

Workout:

Each exercise is performed with given rest time between sets. Complete all sets before advancing to the next exercise. If a resistance feels slightly light, you can change the repetition range to 12-15 instead.

A1 Clean & Jerk – 4x10-12 (per side)

B1 Good Mornings - 3x10-12

B2 Goblet Squats - 3x10-12

C1 Bent Rows - 4x10-12 (per side)

D1 Single Arm Swings - 3x10-12 (per side)

D2 Racked Double Lunges - 3x8 (per side)

Kettlebell Workout Program: Strength-Based Cardio Workout

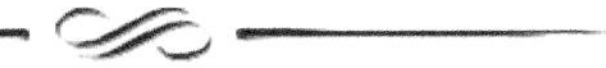

This program will be circuit based, which means you perform an exercise and then move straight into the next exercise with little to no rest. Instead of performing sets, you will be doing rounds instead with several exercises. This is a great workout not just for cardio, but also for when you are limited on time. The entire workout shouldn't last longer than 20-25 minutes if executed properly. Remember to breathe throughout the work and keep oxygen pumping throughout your muscles. It's easy to forget to breathe while focused on intense training, so if you're a trainer this needs to be monitored.

Warm Up (Light Resistance):

A1 Slingshots – 2x8 (per side)

B1 Halos – 2x8 (per side)

C1 Windmill – 2x8 (per side)

Workout:

Remember to complete each exercise and then move on to the next exercise. There are no sets given! You will execute 3-5 rounds depending on athletic levels and ability to complete all exercises.

A1 Cleans - 10-12 (per side)

A2 Push Press - 10-12 (per side)

A3 Single Arm Deadlifts - 10-12 (per side)

A4 Sit and Press – 12-15

A5 Two Handed Swings – 12-15

Kettlebell Workout Program: Core & Mobility Workout

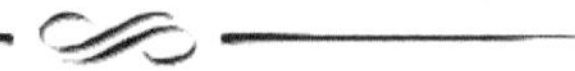

The following workout program is specific to your core and mobility. Your overall intensity level will not be as high, but your muscles are definitely going to be getting activated. Take your time to execute exercises such as the Turkish get up. This was not designed to go at a rapid pace due to the focus needed for your balance. Light to moderate resistance is needed. Anything too heavy may cause injury to the stabilizer muscles that haven't been used very often.

Warm Up (Light Resistance):

A1 Slingshots – 2x8 (per side)

B1 Halos – 2x8 (per side)

C1 Windmill – 2x8 (per side)

Workout

A1 Turkish Get Up – 3-5x3-5 (per side)

B1 Farmer Carry – 3xDistance (per side)

B2 Single Leg Deadlift – 3x10-12 (per side)

C1 Straight Arm Sit Up – 3x8-10 (per side)

D1 Russian Twist – 3x10-12 (per side)

Adding in Additional Exercises

Each workout program is focused on using the kettlebell only. However, you can use kettlebells for a variety of different methods. For example, if you are in a gym you can superset kettlebell swings with cable lat pull downs or seated cable rows. The use of your lats and traps makes this a great fit. On leg days, the kettlebell single leg deadlift is able to superset well with single leg extensions. Cross training was mentioned previously as well for the use of kettlebells. An example of cross training would be performing Turkish get ups for a warm up prior to Olympic lifts, or even performed afterwards with slightly heavier resistance and lower rep ranges.

As for the workouts, you can add in a variety of non-kettlebell exercises such as planks between exercises or jump ropes to end the circuit with. Kettlebells truly are versatile in use, and the benefits from them are endless even if only one or two exercises are utilized each week.

Post Training Active Recovery

If you are new to kettlebell training, you are using a lot of new muscles, and experienced users know that muscles can easily become sore after training. The ballistic nature and use of the core muscles takes a lot of energy away from your body by the end of a workout. The end result is sore muscles that are microscopically damaged and in need of new nutrients to restore energy levels, repair, and grow.

Without protein and other nutrients being consumed following your workout, the body becomes fatigued and possibly uses muscles to repair instead. The protein taken from muscles essentially means that hard work you just put into your workout was really for nothing. The only way to counter this is having an established diet in place.

Aside from nutrition, you also want to help your body recover through active movements. Allowing your sore muscles to relax without movement actually makes it worse. You want blood to flow, bringing nutrients to the muscles throughout your body. An easy way to accomplish this is through static stretching and light dynamic stretching. Static stretches are when you hold a position that stretches your muscles and keeps a joint in that range of motion.

Dynamic stretches are ones where you move your body to get more blood flow and get the joints moving. Static stretches are the best post workout because when held long enough, you're actually telling your muscles to relax actively. Holding a stretch for 20 seconds or longer enables this to occur. Pre workout static stretches should only last 10-15 seconds because you don't want your muscles to relax yet.

The day following your workout would be the same if it's intended for rest. Pull up assist bands come in handy to execute light movements that draw blood flow and get the sore muscles moving. They also work great for doing better stretch work that isn't so easy without them. Is a rest day necessary following kettlebell training? Not necessarily. This depends on your experience level and the intensity of certain muscle groups receiving too much attention. A kettlebell workout like the ones provided makes use of your body as a whole, which means no muscle group was overused. In the beginning, specific areas of your body will feel tense for all that are new to kettlebells. However, as your body develops and gets used to the movement, you will not notice this as much. Being active following a workout, no matter how much experience you have, is the most important concept regardless what type of workout you do.

Closing Remarks

Kettlebells truly do offer a wider range of benefits than any other exercises. You can get a full body workout without having to use more than one or two kettlebells. They have stood the test of time, having been used since ancient Greece to assist athletes to compete with more power and endurance. This simple tool has bounced from country to country and now is recognized for its efficient method of strengthening your body.

The kettlebell is there for nearly all to utilize regardless if it is for home training or within the gym. Having a well-rounded knowledge in the use of kettlebells makes you much more efficient at accomplishing your goals. Just always remember to be humble when using this equipment. It is easy to become injured from using excessive weight and performing the exercises incorrectly. Take the initiative and start incorporating these workouts into your weekly training program while the information is still on your mind!

Thanks for taking the time to read my book. I hope it helped you out in some type of way. If you

are not already please go now and follow me here on FB here

https://www.facebook.com/RichardRobertson40/ or here

on instagram https://www.instagram.com/stayingfitafter40club.

By following me you will receive updates on all of my upcoming books, giveaways, also you

will be the first to get free copies of all of my books.

Never miss another update

You can also follow me here on my Author's Page on Amazon.